KT-415-687

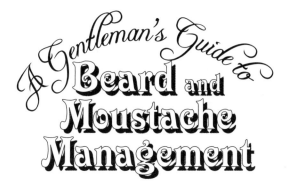

A Gentleman's Guide to Beard and Moustache Management

A Gentleman's Guide to

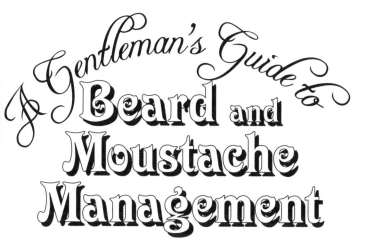

Beard and Moustache Management

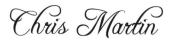

Chris Martin

The
History
Press

With special thanks to the illustrators of this book: Lindsey Smith, for the line drawings in the chapter 'A Guide to Beard & Moustache Styles' and the animal drawings in 'The World of Beards & Moustaches'; and Gwen Burns, for the illustrations in 'A Short History of Facial Hair', 'When Facial Hair Goes Wrong', 'The Hall of Fame' and the depiction of the world's longest beard on p. 149.

First published 2011

Reprinted 2011, 2012, 2013, 2014, 2015

The History Press
The Mill, Brimscombe Port
Stroud, Gloucestershire, GL5 2QG
www.thehistorypress.co.uk

© Chris Martin, 2011

British Library Cataloguing in Publication Data.
A catalogue record for this book is available from the British Library.

ISBN 978 0 7524 5975 2

Typesetting and origination by The History Press
Printed in China.

Contents

☞ **Introduction**   7

☞ **A Short History of Facial Hair**   9

☞ **A Guide to Beard & Moustache Styles**   31

Moustache Styles   34

Beard Styles   54

    Choosing a Shape   55

    Choosing a Style   60

The World Beard & Moustache Championships   78

☞ **When Facial Hair Goes Wrong**   83

Alternatives to the Beard   85

The Worst Facial Hair Ever   90

☞ **The Hall of Fame**   93

Great Moustache Wearers Through History   95

Great Bearded Men Through History   104

☞ **Grooming the Facial Fuzz**   **117**

Essential Equipment   119

Washing & Trimming Beards & Moustaches   125

     Washing your Beard or Moustache   125

     Trimming your Beard or Moustache   126

     Hints & Tips   131

Waxing & Styling   133

Get a Grip: Three Lost Grooming Treasures   138

☞ **The World of Beards & Moustaches**   **141**

Quotes about Beards & Moustaches   143

Beard & Moustache Records   146

Beards & Moustaches in Nature   150

Introduction

THERE IS an old proverb that says it is manners that make a man. While a solid command of your Ps and Qs may cut it during tea with your grandmother, in the real world we all know that facial hair is the true mark of the alpha male.

Beards and moustaches distinguish men from boys and – mercifully – men from women. They create a direct and hot-blooded connection with our dinosaur-wrestling ancestors and demonstrate a dedication to personal style that would leave Beau Brummel speechless.

The *Oxford English Dictionary* defines the verb 'to beard' as 'to boldly confront or challenge someone formidable' and in this book we've done just that. We have defied slovenly convention to raise an overflowing glass to the noble art of pogonotrophy. In these pages you will find beards that define the spirit of adventure and academia that made men great, and moustaches of such sophistication that they could make even the most hard-hearted of ladies swoon.

Whether you favour a French Fork, a Donegal, an American Standard or a Fu Manchu, beards and moustaches – be they waxed or natural – make a powerful statement about the kind of man you are.

We offer you these grooming secrets in the hope of ensuring that a new generation of hirsute gods will walk the earth once more.

A
Short History
of Facial Hair

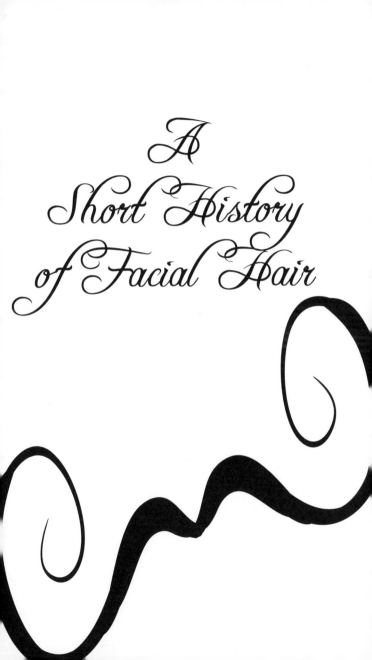

FOR AS long as man has grown facial hair, the beard has been with us. Join us now as we take a journey through the history of pogonotrophy throughout the ages.

PREHISTORIC & NEOLITHIC BEARD MAN

One likes to think that when our earliest ancestors crawled from the primordial ooze, they wore a Goatee at the very least. Our earliest records of the state of men's faces probably come from cave paintings. Unfortunately, the representations of human beings found in these ancient images are usually symbolic, so we don't really know if prehistoric man wore a beard or not. But as these early artists took great care to describe every element of the world around them and there are no drawings of stone razors, mud shaving foam or twig hair tongs, it seems safe to assume that early man was bearded.

Around 300 BC man started shaving with flint. Indeed, archaeologists have found evidence of men using a variety of unpleasant tools to remove their whiskers, including clam shells and sharks' teeth. This must have been extremely tricky and frankly quite painful. Nonetheless, a formal portrait from ancient Iran from around this time shows a man with a magnificent moustache riding a horse while – no doubt – wincing from screaming razor burn.

ANCIENT & CLASSICAL WORLD

In the early classical civilisations we first see the deliberate styling of a man's facial hair, from an unruly and unchecked growth hacked at with sharpened stones, to a refined symbol of manhood, wisdom and prestige.

In the Homeric epics of ancient Greece beards were celebrated and portrayed as a badge of virility. When asking for royal favour, it became a form of entreaty to touch the beard of your king. A smooth face was condemned as a sign of effeminacy to the point where the

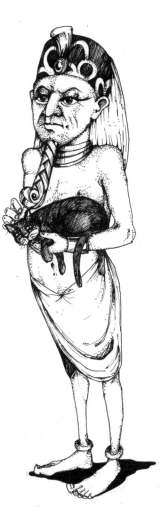

terrifying macho Spartans took to punishing those they considered to be cowards by shaving off their beards.

The ancient Egyptians, on the other hand, were a bit on the fey side and didn't much care for face fuzz. Copper and gold razors used by the pharaohs have been unearthed in Egyptian tombs. While it may have been fashionable to be soft-cheeked, to give the Egyptians their effeminate due they did at least try to enhance the hair they did have on their chins – usually with henna-based dyes or plaits laced with gold thread to show their ranking in society. Ultimately, the only beards that were really valued by the Egyptians were fake ones, and queens, kings and sometimes even sacred cows took to wearing ornate chin covers fashioned from precious metals, known as postiches.

Luckily the two next great civilisations to come along – in Mesopotamia and Persia – were far more in tune with their bearded selves. Their upper classes grew their beards long and took great pains to style them, using special oils and heated tongs to create long patterned tresses and decorative ringlets.

ANCIENT MACEDONIA

Such unchecked growth in the popularity of beards could not continue, and by the time of Alexander the Great it would all go wrong. Legend has it that the Macedonian custom of shaving the face smooth was introduced when Alexander was preparing to fight against the impressively bearded Persians. When one of his officers brought him word that the army was ready for battle, Alexander promptly decreed that all his soldiers be shaved. It has been argued that he feared their beards could be grabbed in combat by their enemies; however, it seems more likely that Alexander – who was just 19 when he became King of Macedonia – probably couldn't grow a beard himself and didn't want to be embarrassed by his hirsute comrades.

Beard-wearers were now faced with a double jeopardy. The first piece of bad news was that this fit of teenage pique was taken seriously by subsequent Macedonian kings and the practice of shaving spread throughout their empire. The second piece of bad news was that the Macedonian empire consisted of the whole

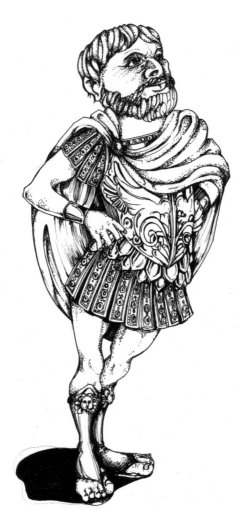

known world. They even passed laws against growing a beard in the great metropolises of Rhodes and Byzantium. The only excluded group was the philosophers, who retained their beards as a badge of their profession – proving without doubt that the stroking of a beard is essential for truly deep thought.

ROME

The Roman Empire would have a laudably hairy start and throughout the period of the Kings of Rome the Romans did not shave. But Pliny tells us that around 299 BC a man named Ticinius brought a barber to Rome, who promptly shaved one of its leading citizens, Scipio Africanus. Africanus must have been something of a trend-setter because the practice seems to have caught on very quickly. After that point a long beard was considered a mark of slovenliness and, oddly enough, foreign tourists.

Soon almost all Roman men were clean-shaven. Traditionally, a Roman would only let his hair and beard grow during mourning. This is the exact opposite to their old rivals, the Greeks, who used to cut off their hair and shave their beards as a display of grief. The association with smelly Greek tourists meant that a smooth face became the sign of being a Roman citizen. In time they even came to consider a bearded man to be 'virtuous and simple'. This sounds good, but in Roman terms it meant you were a pleb.

The need for a close shave meant that barbers' shops became extremely popular in ancient Rome – even the term 'barber' comes from the Latin 'barba', meaning beard. This allowed men who were not wealthy enough to own slaves to pop in for a clean shave on their way to the Forum.

In the latter days of the Roman Republic, decadent and rebellious youth did begin experimenting with facial hair again. Usually they sported partial beards to create an ornamental display. These show beards predictably became a fad in thrill-hungry Rome and prepubescent boys took to oiling their chins in the hope of forcing premature growth.

The first shave a boy took was regarded as the beginning of manhood, and the day on which this took place was celebrated with the hair that was cut off being consecrated to the gods. The emperor and infamous mentalist Nero put his first trim into a golden box set with pearls and dedicated it to Jupiter. Never a great example to anyone, Nero went on to grow one of history's most infamous neck beards and burn Rome to the ground. Historians are unclear whether the two activities were connected.

THE RISE OF THE BARBARIANS

Despite the dominance of the Roman Empire across the world, many other great nations remained unaffected by its vacillations of fashion. In ancient India it has always been no holds barred on the chin rug front. The Indians saw the beard as a symbol of dignity and of wisdom so they let it all hang out – wild and wonderful growths are still worn by *sadhus* and holy men there today. Closer to home in Europe, the Celts grew their hair long and twined it with moustaches that were even longer. One group of Celtic tribes called the Lombards ('Longobards' or 'Langbärte', meaning – you guessed it – long beards) even derived their fame from the great length of their beards.

Meanwhile in the east, the dark forces of the Hunnic Empire were rising. These wild horsemen would sweep across Europe killing everyone in their path as the wind blew through their long, unruly hair.

MIDDLE AGES

The end of the ancient world brought back long hair but introduced a decline in the care of beards, as the newly arriving barbarians valued the ability to kill things far more than personal grooming. Fortunately by the Middle Ages, this devil-may-care combination of hair growth and homicidal skill had been formalised and a proud beard became a symbol of a knight's honour. These new codes of chivalry meant that even so much as touching a knight's beard was a serious offence that could only be sorted out with a bloody duel to the death.

As time passed, Europe saw a return of the preference for shaven faces and smaller beard

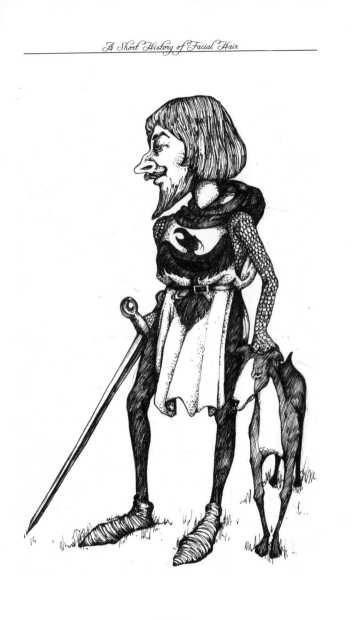

and moustache combinations. Barbers' shops sprung up in medieval cities, but these new high-street entrepreneurs had a slightly different twist on the art of hairdressing than their scissor-wielding Roman predecessors. Medieval barbers also doubled up as surgeons. The traditional red and white barber's pole hung outside the barber's shop was created to symbolise the blood that was associated with such have-a-go surgeries and the bandages that would be required to dress wounds. Basically, the man who shaved you was more likely to pull out your teeth than ask you if you needed something for the weekend. Mercifully this practice ended in the mid-1700s, when surgeons began to focus their skills on medicine and stopped shaving people for cash on the side.

THE RENAISSANCE

In the fifteenth century, European men were largely clean-shaven, but by the sixteenth century beards were back and about to play a key part in a brand new religious war. There were a wide variety of face-dos around at the time, for example the Spanish Spade beard, the English Square-cut beard, the Forked beard and the Stiletto beard (presumably Italian). These beards reflected the foppish and frivolous attitudes of the time. In 1587 such beards entered common speech when – after sending ships to Cadiz, killing hundreds and destroying thirty-seven naval and merchant ships – the lovable licensed pirate Francis Drake claimed that he had singed the King of Spain's beard. What fun!

However, there was nothing fun about the Reformation. It would change the political and religious landscape of the time and reawaken an interest in serious beard growth across Europe. The big beard of a reformer came as a reaction to the Catholic clergymen of the time, who were usually clean-shaven to indicate their celibacy. When a man decided to throw his hat in with the rebellious doctrines of the Protestant Reformation, he would often signal this by allowing his beard to grow. The longer the beard, the more striking the statement – you only need to check out the portraits of John Knox and Thomas Cranmer from the time to see these monster mouth mats in action.

This trend was continued throughout the Catholic Queen Mary's reign, despite it being a time of reaction against Protestant reform, but when Queen Elizabeth I came to the throne she put her foot down. She hated beards and established a tax on them.

By the early seventeenth century beards were once again out of fashion in urban circles of western Europe – and the newly discovered Americas – to such an extent that when Peter the Great of Russia wanted to bring Russian society more in line with the sophisticated west, he ordered men to shave off their beards. He even went so far as to mimic Elizabeth I and levy a tax on beards in 1705. The army, however, remained an exception, and the great popularity of Hussar and Grenadier moustaches meant that soldiers unable to produce this manly decoration were found trying to draw them on with coal.

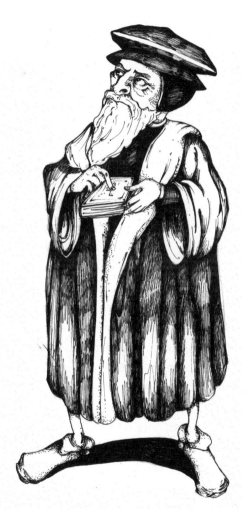

VICTORIAN ERA

The popularity of the beards continued to decline in western society, and by the early eighteenth century most men – particularly amongst the nobility and upper classes – went clean-shaven. There was, however, a dramatic shift in the beard's popularity during the 1850s, when beards were adopted by many kings and emperors, such as Alexander III of Russia, Napoleon III of France and Frederick III of Germany. This royal trend was picked up by leading political and cultural figures, such as Benjamin Disraeli, Charles Dickens, Giuseppe Garibaldi and Giuseppe Verdi. Once again the beard became linked with notions of masculinity and male courage.

Their resulting popularity contributed to some breathtakingly styled ventures in sideburns, beards and moustaches to rival the extraordinary architecture and engineering of the day. It also created the template for the stereotypical Victorian male – a monstrous figure clothed in heavy tweed whose gravitas was indicated by an imposing beard.

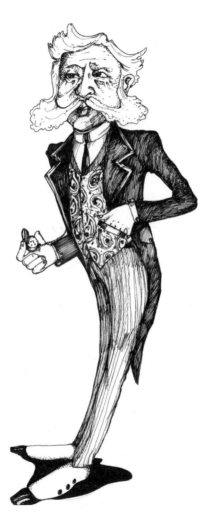

THE MODERN AGE

By the early twentieth century the popularity of beards had begun to wane once again, this time to be replaced by a new enthusiasm for moustaches driven by the rebellious young men of the time. The 1920s and 1930s saw an upsurge in racial political and philosophical thought and with it came challenging moustaches and Goatees worn by the likes of Marcel Proust, Albert Einstein, Vladimir Lenin, Leon Trotsky and Adolf Hitler.

But across the pond, in newly industrialised, post-war America, there were rumblings that would forever change man's relationship with his face fuzz. The development of new shaving technologies – in particular the safety razor and shaving foam in a pressurised tin – meant that for the first time men could enjoy a pain-free shave at home that matched the closeness of a trip to the barber's shop. These advances were further enforced by the development of new advertising and marketing techniques. Indeed, the Gillette Safety Razor Company was one of the first clients of the early advertising titans of

Madison Avenue. Soon, beards and moustaches were vanishing across the western world in favour of clean-shaven faces and business-like crew cuts.

Facial hair was reintroduced to mainstream society by the counterculture of the 1950s and 1960s. The jazz-loving 'beatniks' in the 1950s welcomed back Pencil moustaches, Goatees and Soul Patches, while the anything-goes hippie movement of the mid-1960s completed the revival with everything from full Spade beards to wild and wonderful moustaches. This time it was rock musicians who led the way, with The Beatles, The Byrds, The Beach Boys, and many other bands beginning with 'B', all wearing facial hair.

From the 1980s onwards, the fashion in beards has generally tended towards Goatees, Van Dykes, closely cropped full beards and stubble. In present-day western cultures, the moustache remains sadly quite rare, while in the Middle East and India they are almost compulsory. One thing is noticeable, however: men are no longer tied to one style of facial hair and it has never been easier to chop and change between style to suit your needs, age or mood.

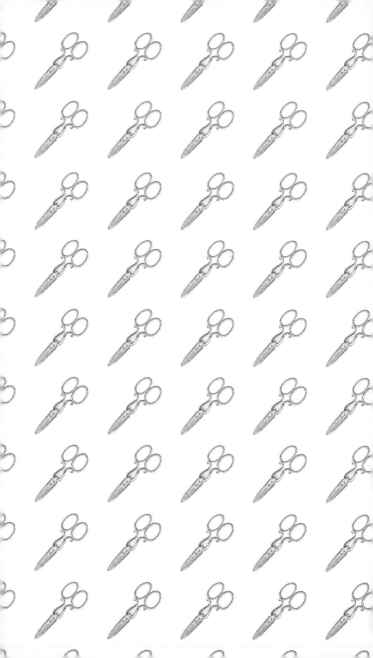

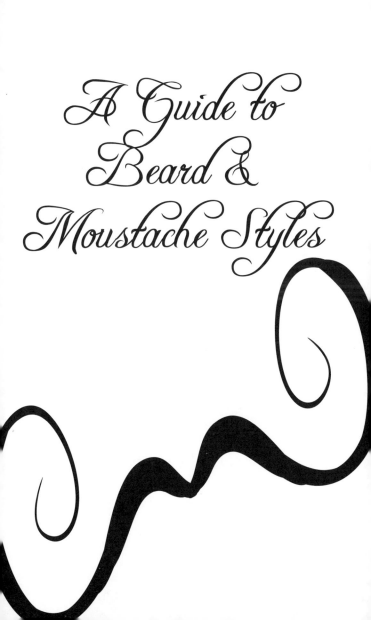

A Guide to
Beard &
Moustache Styles

THE DECISION to grow a beard or moustache is about a lot more than letting yourself go for a few days. It is a living connection with the alpha male gene pool. A hearty beard is the hairy totem of a Neanderthal god and makes its wearer a true lion amongst his fellow men.

While the beard is the mark of man writ large on the cave wall, its companion the moustache is the signature of gent embossed on the heavy business card of his own legend. The world is your oyster when you come to grow a moustache. Throughout history a myriad of different styles have come in and out of fashion, yet each one has symbolised a time and an attitude which can be as relevant today as it was then.

A beard or a moustache is neither an alien invader nor a parasitical companion; it's an outward expression of the inner you, so it is important that once you have made the decision to step back through time and commune with the ancestors, your choice of facial topiary suits both your face and your personality.

MOUSTACHE STYLES

A moustache is a facial statement that reeks of style, individuality and, in some unfortunate cases, soup. When you grow a moustache you're not just covering a prominent overbite or bluffing the fact that you can't afford razor blades, you are making a very public statement about the kind of man you are. As such, it pays to choose wisely.

Below is our guide to the common moustache styles and their hidden meanings.

LEVEL: Amateur Hour ✂

The Chevron

Like hamburgers, muscle cars and pneumatic cheerleaders drunk on Budweiser, the Chevron is an all-American classic. Grown long to cover the top border of the upper lip, this no-nonsense face wedge is worn thick and wide. The perfect compliment to a medallion-adorned barrel chest and diver's watch the size of a dustbin lid, the Chevron doesn't take bullshit from anyone. The Chevron-wearer tells it as he sees it and, yes, he is the kind of man who knows how to handle a woman – which is just like a five iron.

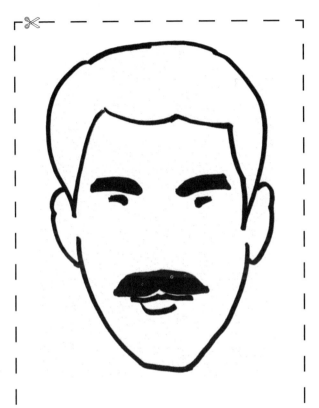

Style yourself on Thomas Magnum (PI).

Try not to look like Ned Flanders.

THE CHEVRON   *Amateur Hour* ✂

The Pencil

Sometimes known as the moth brow, the Pencil is worn narrow and straight and is styled as if drawn on by a pencil. Closely clipped, it creates a mere accent on the upper lip, leaving a scandalously wide shaven gap between the nose and moustache. Widely recognised as the moustache of choice for drug lords, effeminate assassins and ageing tango instructors claiming Jobseeker's Allowance, the Pencil spells out that the wearer has murderous intent – even if it's only on the dance floor.

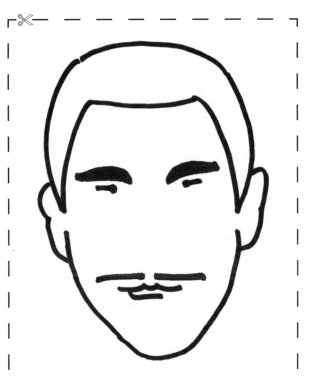

Style yourself on The Artist formerly known as Prince (now known as Prince again).

Try not to look like John Waters.

THE PENCIL   *Amateur Hour*

The Walrus

Delivering exactly what it says on the tin, the Walrus is characterised by a thick, bushy growth of long whiskers that droop over the mouth to give the wearer the appearance of a docile walrus. Once thought to promote good health by shielding the mouth from germs and particles, this monstrous crumb-catcher has proved remarkably popular with philosophers, empire-builders and statesmen over the years – proving once and for all that if something is worth doing, it's worth doing on a massive scale. The Walrus-wearer has an uncontrollable appetite for life to match his uncontrollable appetite for facial hair, which is why you'll find Walrus moustaches littering the faces of great men in history, from Mark Twain to Count Otto Von Bismark.

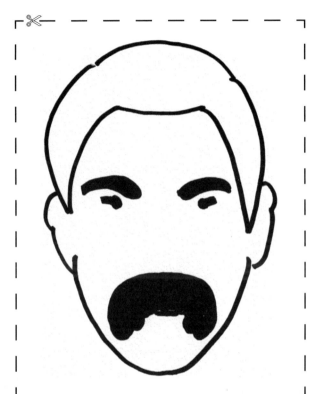

Style yourself on Rudyard Kipling.

Try not to look like David Crosby.

THE WALRUS   *Amateur Hour* ✂

The Mexican

Sometimes known as the 'Pancho Villa' after the crazed Mexican revolutionary of the same name, this monster soup-strainer is worn big, bold and bushy. It's an unruly growth of hair beginning from the middle of the upper lip and pulled roughly to the sides to provide just enough space to insert the neck of a Tequila bottle. The Mexican is a two-statement moustache. The first of those statements is 'I don't own a pair of scissors'; the second is 'I'm going to raze your village to the ground'. Accessorise this baby with a two-day growth of stubble on the chin.

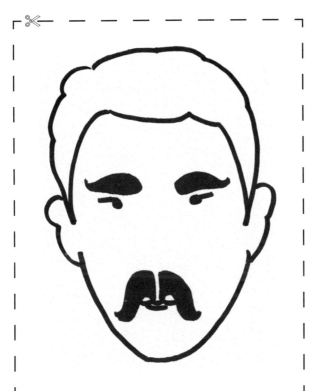

Style yourself on Cheech Marin.

Try not to look like Yosemite Sam.

THE MEXICAN   *Amateur Hour* ✂

LEVEL: Semi-Pro ✂<✂<

The Horseshoe

Designed for the real man, the Horseshoe is a full moustache with vertical extensions grown down the sides of the mouth to the jaw line to resemble an upside-down U. The whiskers running along the sides of the mouth are sometimes referred to as the 'pipes'. The Horseshoe says a million different things about the wearer and all of them are bad. A perennial favourite of convicts, bikers and off-duty special forces operatives the world over, wearing this moustache makes it clear you're the kind of man who likes to settle his problems with a bottle of Jack Daniels and a broken pool cue.

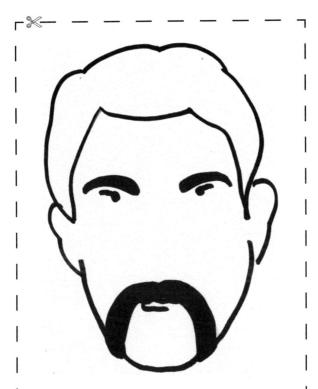

Style yourself on Lemmy Kilmister from Motörhead.

Try not to look like Derek Smalls from Spinal Tap.

THE HORSESHOE

Semi-Pro ✄✄

The Handlebar

A classic Handlebar moustache can be worn large or small (the 'Petit Handlebar'). It is grown bushy and long enough to curl the ends skyward with the aid of styling wax to resemble a set of fruity bicycle handlebars. The Handlebar moustache combines dignity, sophistication and an air of flamboyant rebellion with a set of easy-to-grasp-and-twiddle ends for use while announcing evil plans. It's no surprise that this classic tash is beloved of eccentrics the world over. So if you're cloning an army of gas-powered super soldiers in an underground laboratory or simply creating a OO gauge replica of the *Flying Scotsman* in your garden shed, the Handlebar is for you.

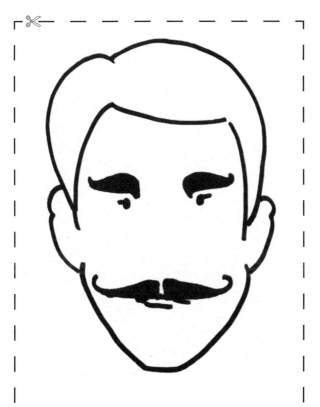

Style yourself on Jimmy Edwards.

Try not to look like Super Mario.

THE HANDLEBAR   *Semi-Pro* ✂✂

The English

The sun may have set on the British Empire but the moustache that built it lives on. The English is a narrow, divided moustache that begins at the middle of the upper lip with its long whiskers pulled to either side of the centre, and it reeks of blue-blooded class. The areas beyond the corners of the mouth are typically shaved because you're a cad, you're a bounder and you probably fly to work in a Spitfire. The English tells the world you inherited this moustache from your father (along with his 400-acre farm in Gloucestershire and his flatulent, ageing Labrador), and by God you look good in it.

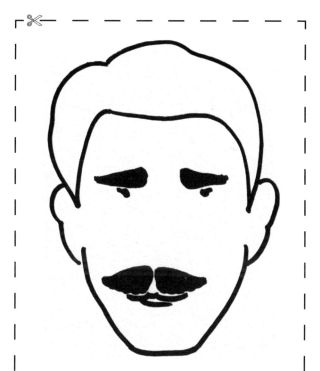

Style yourself on Terry Thomas.

Try not to look like Dick Dastardly.

THE ENGLISH   *Semi-Pro* ✂✂

LEVEL: Don't Try This At Home ><><><

The Toothbrush

The Toothbrush moustache has a baffling variety of names: the Charlie Chaplin, the 1/3, the Philtrum, the Postage Stamp or the Soul Moustache. It is a thick growth shaved to be about an inch wide and worn in the centre of the lip. The style is said to have originated in 1920s Germany, as working-class men responded to the flamboyant moustaches of the upper classes with a new brand of clipped, focused lip wear. Unfortunately, one of those working-class men was Adolf Hitler and the moustache – like the Third Reich – would become deeply unpopular after 1945. Nowadays this practical, minimalist tash is not for the faint-hearted. Sported solely by African dictators, psychotic eighties' synth players and those looking to pick a fight at a Girl Guides' tea party, it's best left to the professionals.

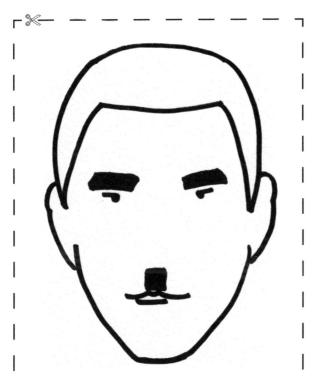

Style yourself on Oliver Hardy.

Try not to look like Robert Mugabe.

THE TOOTHBRUSH   *Don't Try This At Home* ✂✂✂

Fu Manchu

For centuries a closely guarded secret of the mysterious court of the Chinese emperors, it took an exploitative and wildly racist 1923 movie to bring the Fu Manchu to prominence in the west. This infamous moustache is worn thin and straight. Grown downwards past the lips, it extends towards tapered ends which hang low to complete far below the chin. This tash differs from the Horseshoe in its evil elegance and – as it is only grown from the upper lip – because its sides remain enigmatically shaved. The Fu Manchu is an outward expression of a deviant intelligence bent on world domination and the control of men's minds through bribery, sorcery and lingering inscrutable stares. As such, The Fu Manchu is easier to carry off in a vastly ornate imperial palace or smoky Shanghai opium den than while fighting for a seat on a crowded commuter train into Charing Cross.

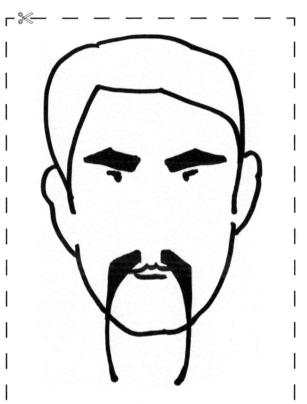

Style yourself on Anton LaVey.

Try not to look like Ming the Merciless.

FU MANCHU   *Don't Try This At Home* ✂✂✂

The Dali

Salvador Dali lived his life as art, so it was no surprise that his extraordinary facial statement was subsequently named after him. The Dali is more a piece of art than a moustache. Strictly it should be created only from narrow points of hair originating on the lower lip, which are bent or curved steeply upwards on either side of the nose while leaving all other areas around the mouth shaved. Artificial styling aids are a must to defy both gravity and the shackles of convention. This style was just the tip of the iceberg for Dali, and the great Catalan artist even published a book of variations featuring the moustache customised with flowers, horns and bows. The wearer becomes the artist in the creation of a Dali – which is just as well, as a tub of styling wax is around £150,000 cheaper than one of Dali's paintings.

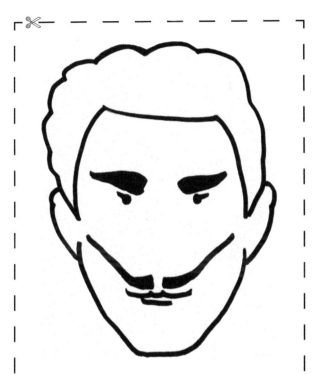

Style yourself on Salvador Dali (who else?).

Try not to look like a nutter.

THE DALI   *Don't Try This At Home* ✂✂✂

BEARD STYLES

While a moustache may be about style, panache and something that looks good with the fancy cigarette holder you got for Christmas, a beard is all about the testosterone.

For its uncompromising power and disturbing ability to take on a life of its own, the king of all men's beard styles must surely be a full-face number that hangs from the face like animal pelt. But the truth is that the full-face beard is not always possible to grow for some men or a desirable option for others. Luckily, for those of us who have a weak disposition, a job they want to keep or just lacklustre follicles, there are a multitude of beard styles each as dramatic and imposing as a polar bear with an Uzi.

Plus, there's the added bonus that some correctly styled face fuzz can go a long way to enhance the features you are most proud of, while masking your weaker points. In short, a well-appointed beard can make a young man look older and more rugged, and an old, fat man look half his age and size.

Here is our guide to choosing the right rug for your mug.

A Word on Large & Small Faces

Whatever the shape of your face, you'll also need to consider the size of your head. If you have a large face then you'll need to have a beard to match, a short style will simply make your head look huge – keep the beard full and the moustache wide.

Conversely, if you a have a small face, resist the urge to get carried away with your whiskers or you'll end up looking like a pan scrubber with two eyes stuck on it. In both cases you will need to follow the rules listed below on styles that are appropriate to individual face shapes.

Choosing a Shape

Having established the size of your head, the shape of your face is the next factor in choosing a beard. Below are some basic dos and don'ts for face shapes.

Round Faces

If you have a round face, look for a style that is full and long on the chin to add length to your face and make it appear less round. Keep the sides of the beard close or shaved, and watch the length of your sideburns if you don't want to end up looking like a sunflower.

Long Faces

You can also use your beard to shorten your face. Those with long faces will require a beard which is fuller at the sides and shorter on the chin. Again, you're using your whiskers to change the shape of your face to make it appear less long.

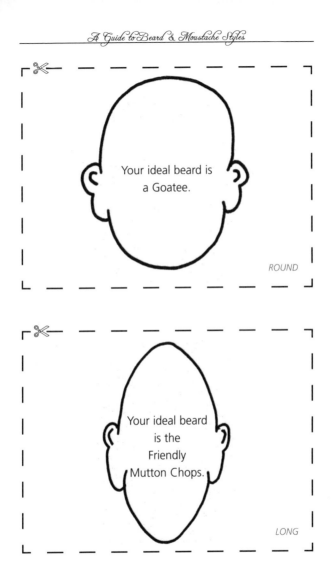

Your ideal beard is
a Goatee.

ROUND

Your ideal beard
is the
Friendly
Mutton Chops.

LONG

Square Faces

Similar to shaping a beard for a round face, the beard for a square face should be shorter at the sides and longer at the chin to add length to the face. However, you can further enhance the effect by trimming or styling your chin hair into a stylish point.

Oval Face

Hallelujah! If you have an oval face then you've lucked out as the oval is considered the Holy Grail of face shapes when it comes to growing a beard – you can wear anything, my friend. However, with all the styles suggested here, make sure the various lengths of your whiskers are blended together to achieve a natural appearance or you'll look like you've trimmed your pride and joy with a set of garden shears.

Your ideal beard is the
Ducktail or the Anchor.

SQUARE

Your ideal beard is
whatever you like,
it'll all look good.

OVAL

Choosing a Style

The Chinstrap

The Chinstrap or Chin Curtain covers a wide variety of styles based around a full beard with the moustache and chin shaved. Usually this involves long sideburns which connect under the chin to create a strap effect running from one side of the face to the other. If you want to look like you've escaped from an Amish community then grow the hair full and let it creep over the chin – this is also known as the Donegal. Trim your whiskers to a pencil-thin line under the chin and you've got yourself the classic Douche Bag beard, inexplicably beloved of hammer-headed American high school students. Most men can grow hair on the chin and neck even when they haven't yet developed the ability to force it out on the top lip, so it's no surprise that the Chinstrap in its various forms has proven perennially popular with younger people.

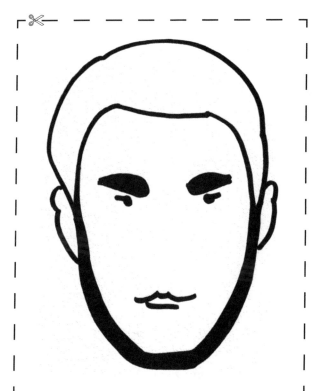

Style yourself on Abraham Lincoln.

Try not to look like Fred Durst.

THE CHINSTRAP   *Amateur Hour* ✂

The Goatee

A Goatee is a thick tuft of hair grown on the chin, sometimes rising to meet the corners of the mouth, so called because it makes you look like a goat. It's commonly associated with students, pseudo-intellectuals and the bass players of unsigned indie bands. The Goatee says: 'I'm so much of a rebel, I don't even have a conventional beard!' It's a style which could only be designed to impress prepubescent girls and depress your mother – as a result, the beard and the bad-ass attitude it conveys really shouldn't be touted around outside of your twenties or you'll end up looking like an ageing A&R man with three ex-wives and a raging coke habit. The Goatee is a good look but it has its place and shouldn't be a lifelong commitment. Enjoy it while you can.

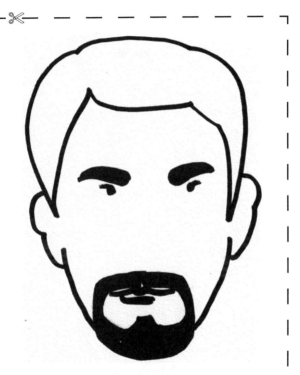

Style yourself on Leonardo DiCaprio.

Try not to look like Shaggy from
Scooby Doo.

THE GOATEE   *Amateur Hour* ✂

Stubble

This is essentially a very short beard of a few days' growth that only became formalised as a style when it became inexplicably fashionable during the 1980s. Then known as 'Designer Stubble', it was synonymous in popular culture with Don Johnson, George Michael and the first three *Die Hard* movies. Indeed, this look was so associated with TV detective Sonny Crockett that one resourceful character actually marketed a trimmer called the Miami Device. You will need an electric trimmer to manage your stubble as only a trimmer will allow you to crop it to a pre-set length – to shave to achieve the effect of not shaving, basically. Whether it actually counts as a beard or as just the by-product of a late night is debatable, but it's certainly a great way of getting the feel of facial hair without making too much of a commitment.

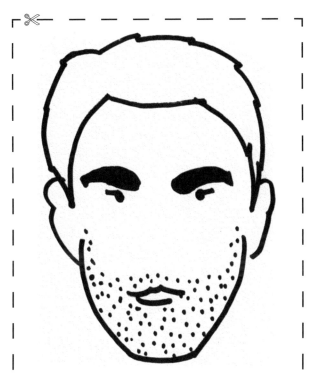

Style yourself on David Beckham.

Try not to look like Serge Gainsbourg.

STUBBLE   *Amateur Hour*

LEVEL: Semi-Pro ⸓<⸓<

The Van Dyke

However it is styled, the Van Dyke is a beard for people with artistic pretensions who like to express their creativity through the medium of human hair. Named after the seventeeth-century Flemish painter Anthony van Dyck, the Van Dyke is technically just a Goatee accompanied by a moustache, with the hair on the cheeks shaven. But the Van Dyke is also a catch-all for a wide grouping of beard styles that are made up from this classic moustache and long Goatee combo. Popular variants include a luxurious curled moustache above a dangling Soul Patch channelling Wild Bill Hickock to a pencil-thin perv tash floating over a squared-off chin box like Dave Navarro. To give it its due, the Van Dyke does hold a certain air of tragic mystery. As a result it has managed to become a staple of magicians, mind readers and evil-looking Latin teachers worldwide.

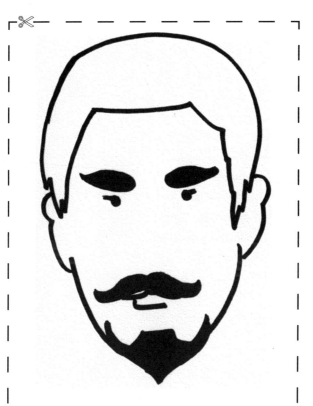

Style yourself on Johnny Depp.

Try not to look like Colonel Sanders.

THE VAN DYKE   Semi-Pro ✂✂

The Ducktail, Hollywoodian, Anchor, Royale & Balbo

As we have already noted, there are a myriad of styles based around the combination of moustache and Goatee. You are only really constrained by the need to shave your cheeks and neck and by the limits your own imagination. Wear your moustache bushy with a trimmed, pointed Goatee and you've got a Ducktail. Square that Goatee off and you've got a Hollywoodian. Wear a thin moustache that follows the line of the mouth with a wide, thick beard and you've got a Balbo. Trim that moustache and Goatee further to create an anchor. Whichever style you choose to go with, it is inevitable that you will eventually end up at the same place – that place where you are possessed with an uncontrollable desire to let both beard and moustache grow long so you can style the tips into fabulous tapered points, because that luxurious, flamboyant beard is the beard of kings and conquerors, and is known simply as the Royale.

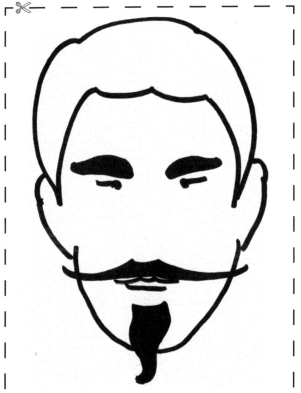

Style yourself on Robert De Niro.

Try not to look like Catweazle.

THE DUCKTAIL, HOLLYWOODIAN, ANCHOR, ROYALE & BALBO

Semi-Pro ✂✂

The Soul Patch

Seldom has so little said so much to so many – the Soul Patch (also known as a Mouche) is a small patch of facial hair just below the lower lip and above the chin. Coming to beatnik prominence in the 1950s and 1960s, where it became popular with jazzmen, writers and other subversive arty types, it's still the facial adornment of choice for ageing rock stars and those who live in a shed in a far corner of the left field. Combine it with a generous manicured moustache and you have a powerful look that says you're a lady killer who knows his way around a box of watercolours. One word of warning, though – the solo Soul Patch will draw general disdain from beard haters and sceptics everywhere. Indeed, HRH the Duke of Edinburgh – a clean-shaven man not known for his tact – commented on first seeing one: 'If you are going to grow a beard, grow a beard.' He may have had a point.

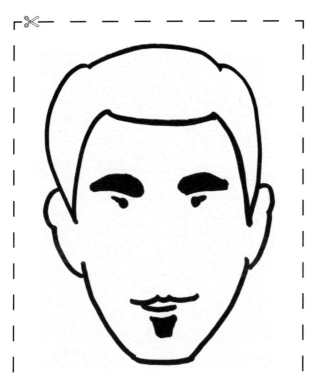

Style yourself on Frank Zappa.

Try not to look like Geddy Lee.

THE SOUL PATCH   Semi-Pro ✂✂

LEVEL: Don't Try This At Home ><><><

Mutton Chops

A favourite with blustering red-faced Victorians and late-night visitors to Soho, Mutton Chops are bushy sideburns grown across the cheeks in the shape of a lamb chop with a shaved chin. They go hand in hand with the Friendly Mutton Chops, which add a connected moustache to the look. Really more of an out-of-control sideburn than a beard, their practical application has meant they are widely associated with two key user groups. The first is the military (the name Sideburn was coined for the American Civil War General Ambrose Burnside, who sported a magnificent pair), who used the thick hair to protect their cheeks from powder burns while firing muskets. Ironically, the military would also instigate the Mutton Chops' fall from popularity when they worked out that such sideburns spoiled the seal on a gas mask and switched to moustaches. The second is the gay community, which has resulted in this style also being known as 'bugger grips' – though it seems unlikely they have ever been used for this purpose.

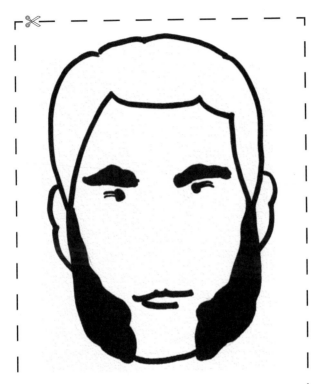

Style yourself on Wolverine.

Try not to look like Noddy Holder.

MUTTON CHOPS   *Don't Try This At Home* ✂✂✂

Full Beard

The Full Beard is the classic expression of the male beard. A Full Beard says: 'I am a man, I am confident, handsome, and I live in a cave in the mountains where I kill and eat wolves.' Covering the whole face, it comprises a long, thick growth of downward-flowing whiskers on the cheeks and chin with either a styled or integrated moustache of similar girth. The trick to rocking a Full Beard is to define its shape. You can do this by squaring or rounding off the chin hair and cutting a regular cheek and neck line to provide some clear borders. But don't cut the cheek line too low or you'll neuter the breathtaking impact of this monster. A Full Beard is a sign of wisdom and erudition, so it's no surprise that you'll find it adorning the visages of some of the most influential men in history, notably Moses, Karl Marx and Charles Darwin.

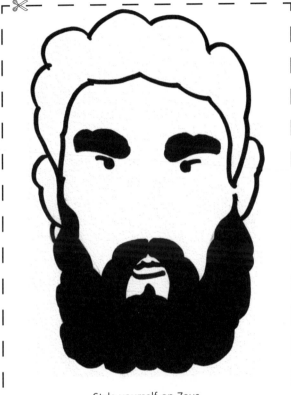

Style yourself on Zeus.

Try not to look like Billy Gibbons from ZZ Top.

FULL BEARD   *Don't Try This At Home* ✂✂✂

The Neck Beard

The Neck Beard or 'Neard' is similar to the Chinstrap but with the chin and jaw line shaven to leave a slightly unusual growth of hair on the neck alone. This particular beard hasn't really been popular for over a century, as it is – frankly – rather an odd thing to do. Those who wear it have usually been a bit psycho, notably the Emperor Nero and Horace Greeley, who blew his fortune on fake diamonds, went mad and ran one of the least successful presidential campaigns in history. This is definitely one for enthusiasts only.

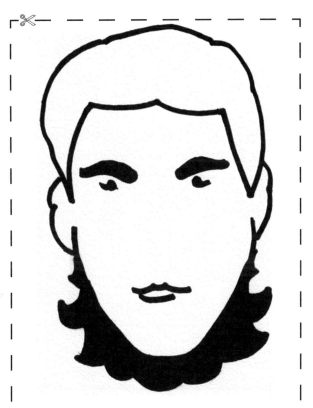

Style yourself on Richard Wagner.

Try not to look like Henry David Thoreau.

THE NECK BEARD   *Don't Try This At Home* ✂✂✂

THE WORLD BEARD & MOUSTACHE CHAMPIONSHIPS

It would be impossible to write about the art of pogonotrophy without taking a moment to pay tribute to the biennial congregation of facial hair enthusiasts and all-round mentalists that is known as the World Beard & Moustache Championships.

First held in Höfen-Enz, Germany, the event brings together hundreds of men with beards and moustaches who enter their highly styled facial hair into the merciless ring of world-class competition. Since its inception in 1990, the event has been held in the UK, the United States and Sweden. The most recent event, which was held in Anchorage, Alaska, in 2009, boasted the highest ever attendance and raised over $16,000 for charity.

Aside from the sterling role the championships play in the promotion of facial hair and its awesome creative possibilities, they also serve to properly define the modern facial hair landscape. There are three groups of growth recognised by the competition: Moustache, Partial Beard and

Full Beard, with each section being broken down into individual classes.

Moustache

Natural Moustache – Growth of a maximum of 1.5cm beyond the end of the upper lip, which may be styled (but without aids).

English – Slender growth which is extremely long and pulled to the side.

Dali – Slender growth with long tips, straight up or arching up.

Imperial – Small and bushy growth with tips arching up.

Hungarian – Big and bushy growth, beginning from the middle of the upper lip and pulled to the side.

Moustache Freestyle – Any moustache that does not match the other classes.

Partial Beard

Natural Goatee – Facial hair grown only on the chin, upper and lower lip, which may be styled (but without aids).

Chinese – Chin shaved with moustache tips grown long and pulled down.

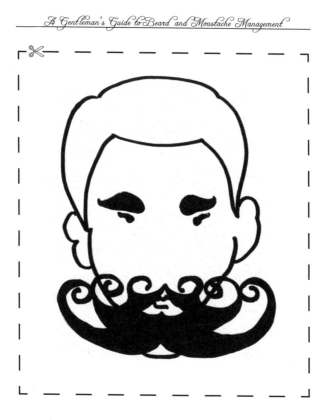

Musketeer – Moustache grown long and slender above a small and pointed beard.

Imperial – Hair of any length grown only on the cheeks and upper lip.

Sideburns Freestyle – Sideburns with shaved chin.

Alaskan Whaler – Any beards with no moustache.

Partial Beard Freestyle – Any partial beard that does not match the other classes.

Full Beard

Verdi – Short and round growth where length does not exceed 10cm.

Garibaldi – Broad, full and round growth where length does not exceed 20cm.

Natural Full Beard – Grown as desired and styled (but without aids).

Natural Full Beard with Styled Moustache – Grown as desired but only the moustache can be styled (but without aids).

Full Beard Freestyle – Any full beard that does not match the other classes.

The current world champion is a 33-year-old Alaskan. David Traver beat 140 competitors to win the first prize in the freestyle beard category, with 20.5 inches of curled facial hair in the shape of a snowshoe. Tragically, the current champion will not be defending his coveted title at the 2011 championships in Trondheim, Norway, as he gallantly offered to shave off his award-winning chin rug for charity.

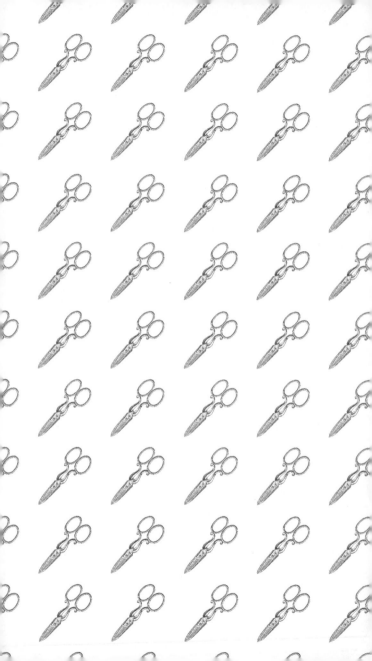

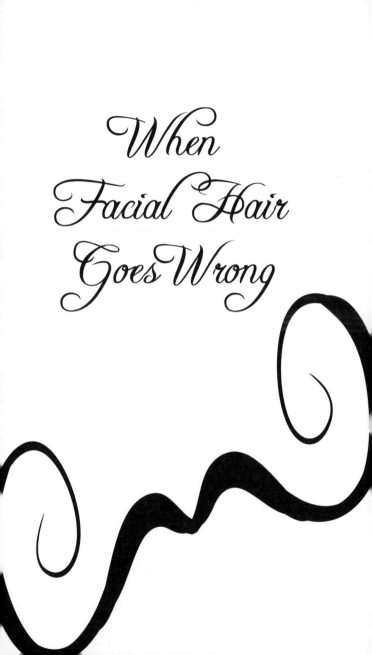

When
Facial Hair
Goes Wrong

FOR MOST men, a beard or moustache serves as a fast track to an exciting new world of possibilities, but for some unfortunate others it's little more than a gateway to hell. Whether you think you're setting a trend or trying to get away with some anorexic tufts that make you look like a teenage virgin, get it wrong and you'll become a laughing stock among friends and family alike.

The road is long and hard for those with stupid or ill-judged facial hair and it is walked alone. Don't say we didn't warn you.

ALTERNATIVES TO THE BEARD

When you've finally made the momentous decision to grow some face fungus, it can be a bitter disappointment to discover that you haven't got the follicular fortitude to carry it through. In most cases, the unfortunate smooth-faced soul will accept their lot, but many others simply cannot live with the fact and have recourse to some extreme solutions. We don't recommend you try any of these, but below are listed some of the wild and wonderful alternatives attempted by those left bereft by their lack of facial lawn.

Falsies

The ancient Egyptians wore ornate metal beards; the Elizabethans sometimes wore facial wigs; and many a misguided individual has tried to get away with drawing on a moustache and beard with face paints, coal and even the school nativity favourite, cocoa. Take our advice, if you are going to wear a false beard, wait for Christmas and get a job in Santa's Grotto at Debenhams – it's the only way you'll be taken seriously wearing one.

Face Chains

Is it jewellery or is it a metal beard? This is the question that no one will be asking as you rattle into your local pub. Face chains were a new type of jewellery designed by Spaniard Carlos Diez for the 2008 Pasarela Cibeles show in Madrid. They were created from long chains suspended from the ears that hung from the face below the nose in interlinked patterns. Allegedly influenced by S&M, they have – unsurprisingly – failed to catch on.

Lotions & Potions

Throughout history people have sought to promote hair growth through advances in medical science and less formal home remedies they believe will help them along. Even today some swear by a bizarre cocktail of unguents – olive oil, steroid cream and Rogaine spring to mind. However, playing chemist on the sensitive skin of your face is extremely ill advised and frankly ineffective.

Balaclava Beards

Another alternative was provided by the world of wacky fashion when designer Vík Prjónsdóttir decided to create a twist to the already perfectly functional balaclava by adding a knitted moustache and beard. On the one hand they're warm and you get to wear a balaclava without looking like you're about to rob a bank. On the other, these woollen monstrosities – which come in a choice of styles like 'Lumberjack', 'Viking' and 'Pirate' – are just ridiculous.

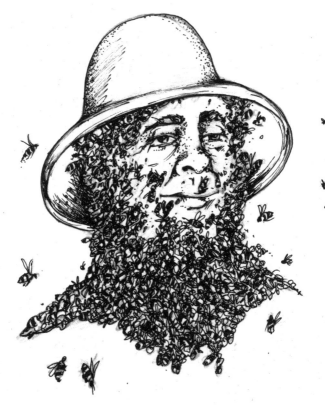

Bearded Underwear

Originally dreamed up by French artist Ephinia, the bearded brief was – allegedly – a retort to male machismo. Entitled 'Sex Bomb', referring to the bomb drawn on the backside, the lead creation in the collection featured the face of Osama Bin Laden with a long beard trailing between the wearer's thighs. Other briefs available included 'Family Jewels', 'A Nest for a Small Bird' and 'Elite Shooter'. Seriously, facial hair is meant for the face. Steer well clear.

Beard of Bees

Bee bearding is the frankly insane practice of wearing several thousand honey bees on your face. Bees are actually quite emotionally sensitive creatures and traditionally, beekeepers have allowed bees to rest on their bodies in order to build up a rapport with them. However, it took a Russian mentalist called Peter Prokopovitch to perfect the art of fashioning a rudimentary beard from them in the 1830s. The 'beard' is achieved by strapping a small cage containing a queen bee under the chin. It is her charms that draw the crowd to form your mobile apiary. But take note: bee bearding is not for the faint-hearted. Bee beards are not rated by size or style but weight, with the current world record being held by American animal trainer Mark Biancaniello. He wore 350,000 bees, weighing just over 87lb, during a 1998 broadcast of the *Guinness World Records* TV show.

Beard Bags

You want a beard but also need a bag? Caroline Ballhorn's felt and vinyl Beard Bags have managed to cover both bases. A beard bag is basically a totally unrealistic hollow beard that is attached to the face by hooks over the ears. And you had better have strong ears, because once you've filled it with your cards, house keys, mobile and other sundry items, it's going to weigh a ton.

THE WORST FACIAL HAIR EVER

Frida Kahlo

Frida Kahlo was a Mexican artist of the 1940s and 1950s. Best known for her colourful and imposing self-portraits, Kahlo's art was admired for its ability to capture the inner pain and passion of her subject and was latterly celebrated for its uncompromising examination of the female experience – which is an art critic's shorthand for saying that in both life and art Kahlo had a bloody great tash and her eyebrows joined in the middle. While it is difficult to say whether Kahlo's self-portraits would have been less successful had she shaved, they would certainly have been less disturbing to look at.

Bearded Ladies

A lady may find herself with a beard as the result of hormonal imbalance, a rare genetic disorder known as hypertrichosis, or maybe just by being a Russian weightlifter on too many anabolic steroids – either way, growing a beard if you are a lady is wrong. No ifs. No buts. It's wrong. Almost every culture in the world pressures women to remove their beards and – outside of a circus sideshow – growing a beard will certainly be viewed as a social stigma. Don't do it.

And Finally … Brad Pitt's Beard

Most women would agree that Brad Pitt is one of the sexiest men alive. Just being good looking would have been enough for most men, but Brad is also photogenic, hard-bodied, famous and rich beyond the wildest dreams of Croesus. Did we also mention that he's going out with one of the world's most beautiful women and has four equally attractive kids? Luckily for us normal guys, Brad's seemingly perfect life went badly wrong when he tried to grow a beard. First he tried it long and straggly and ended up looking like a wet dog, then he moved on to a hideous grey French Fork, before finally settling – heaven forbid – on a Goatee adorned with *Pirates of the Caribbean*-style trinkets. Brad got it wrong – badly wrong.

The Hall of Fame

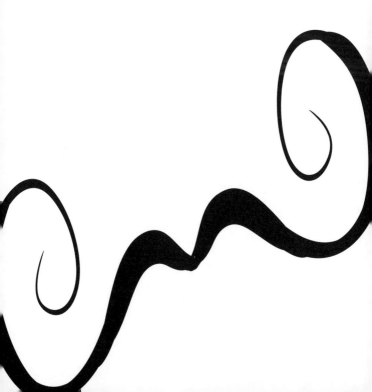

WHETHER IT be a full Spade beard that strikes silent awe into a crowded lecture theatre or a pencil-thin lip line that can drop a lady's knickers at fifty paces, beards and moustaches have been with us since the dawn of time. So it's no surprise that some of the greatest men in history have been defined by – and have come to define – their choice of facial adornment.

GREAT MOUSTACHE WEARERS THROUGH HISTORY

Charlie Chaplin

Chaplin was a screen god of the silent era and one of the greatest movie stars of all time. He made over eighty films in his life – in most cases starring, writing, directing and even scoring them himself. While Chaplin often went smooth-shaven off screen, he is inextricably linked with the Toothbrush moustache that he created for his most famous character, the Tramp. The tash was whimsical and comic, and above all easy to draw on with greasepaint. This clipped style became synonymous with Chaplin, endearing the multi-talented actor to his millions of fans and helping to distract the US government from his communist leanings and a lifelong enthusiasm for underage girls.

The Biker from the Village People

For three magical years, the insanely catchy music of the Village People ruled the air waves and dance floors of the world. The group's selling point was their on-stage costumes which depicted American cultural stereotypes in a not-at-all camp way. For most of the group the stage was where the dressing up ended, but it was not so for 'The Biker', aka Glenn M. Hughes, whose persona became a rugged way of life. Hughes' powerful bass voice was an important part of the Village People's sound, but his greatest contribution was surely his extravagant Horseshoe moustache and trademark leather outfit. Hughes even became a biker in real life and kept a shiny Harley Davidson parked outside his home. It just goes to prove that you can't fake it when it comes to wearing a serious tash.

Burt Reynolds

'What I look for mostly in a man is humour, honesty and a moustache. Burt has all three,' said the actress Sally Field, summing up the genius of Burt Reynolds. And what a moustache it was; few people can claim to own their lip caterpillar in the way that Burt Reynolds does. The American actor is as synonymous with the macho, all-action Standard he wears on his top lip as he is with low-grade action comedies and high-profile bankruptcies. Sat smugly between Burt's pearly white teeth and his surgically altered nose, the moustache is one of America's most recognisable pieces of facial hair. Burt's 'mo' has starred in more than ninety feature films and 300 television episodes.

Clark Gable

Best known for playing Rhett Butler in the Civil War epic *Gone with the Wind*, the film actor Clark Gable was known as the 'King of Hollywood' in his heyday. A three-time Oscar nominee, he was one of the greatest leading men of all time. During his long career, Gable appeared opposite some of the most prolific leading actresses and effortlessly bedded most of them. Part of his appeal had to have been the rakish Pencil moustache he wore throughout his stellar career: sophisticated without being sleazy; refined without being effeminate. Gable wore his tash like it had been designed for him and the ladies loved it. His long-time friend, co-star and on-off romance Joan Crawford, said of Gable: 'he was a king wherever he went. He walked like one, he behaved like one, and he was the most masculine man that I have ever met in my life.' I wonder if she would have said the same had he had a Neck Beard.

Frank Zappa

Frank Zappa was an avant-garde composer, singer-songwriter and record producer. Across his thirty-year career, Zappa produced an incredible sixty jazz, electronic and orchestral albums – a body of work that identified him as an absolutely unique musician working on the experimental fringes of music. Though Zappa lived through untold changes in music fashion, from psychedelia to punk rock, he remained true to his convictions musically and in his choice of facial hair. Throughout it all he sported his trademark droopy Mexican moustache combined with a vibrant Soul Patch – a look that became so resonant of the man that this off-beat combination could arguably be renamed 'The Zappa'.

Mark Spitz

Long before Michael Phelps was old enough to load his own bong, American swimmer Mark Spitz had won seven gold medals at a single Olympic games. Spitz's achievement crowned a career that had already seen him named World Swimmer of the Year in 1969, 1971 and 1972, and he did it all from behind a globally famous moustache. Spitz originally grew the tash because his coach had bet the teenage swimmer that he couldn't. In a sport where the athletes usually shaved off all their body hair to decrease drag, Spitz's unique cookie duster became intrinsically linked with his world-beating sporting prowess. When quizzed about the 'mo' by the Russian coach, Spitz claimed that the crumb-catcher created a pocket of air to help him breathe and that its shape acted like a plough that cut through the water. Even though Spitz had been joking, the

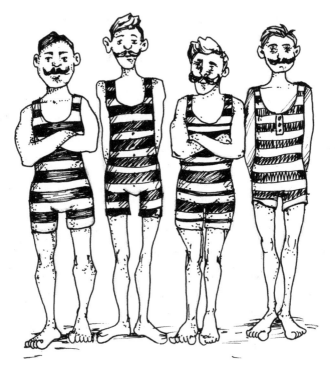

Russians took him at face value and the following year the entire Russian swim team turned up with matching tashes.

George Armstrong Custer

Despite being one of the United States' most famous cavalry commanders, the life of George Armstrong Custer was something of a failure. He graduated last from his class at West Point, was demoted from major-general to captain at the end of the Civil War and was once court-martialled for going absent without leave. Custer was considering alternative careers when he signed up to serve in the Indian Wars of the 1870s. Here he barely had time to get a couple of massacres under his belt before it all came to a sticky end at the Battle of Little Bighorn. But where Custer did achieve great success was in the facial hair department. His trademark combination of long flowing locks and a generous droopy moustache captured the public's imagination and ensured his immortality in folklore and historically vague Wild West shows for all time.

Friedrich Nietzsche

Friedrich Wilhelm Nietzsche was a nineteenth-century German philosopher who sported an untamed Walrus moustache to match the wild ambition of his thought. As Nietzsche produced critical texts on religion, morality, contemporary culture, philosophy and science, the moustache took on a life of its own, eventually growing into the bushy monster that made him the envy of his faculty at the University of Basel. In philosophical terms, Nietzsche's influence remains substantial. Central to his thought was the idea of life-affirmation, which involves an honest questioning of all doctrines that deplete life's energies. He seems to have also applied this credo to his face as, by the age of 24, his tash was well out of control. Sadly, the brighter the candle, the shorter its life. Nietzsche would spend his latter years battling mental illness and tertiary syphilis in the care of his family.

Lord Kitchener

To most of us, he is best known as the poster boy of the First World War, whose stern demeanour entreated the young men of Britain to die in a variety of hideous ways in the waist-deep mud of the French countryside. Yet Field Marshal The Rt Hon. Sir Horatio Herbert Kitchener, 1st Earl Kitchener KG, KP, GCB, OM, GCSI, GCMG, GCIE, ADC, PC, was a British soldier who was already nationally famous for his campaigns across the British Empire in Palestine, Sudan, Egypt, South Africa and India. Throughout his life, Kitchener wore what is probably the last of the great Victorian nose caterpillars: 14ft wide, as big as your arm and waxed rigid enough to withstand a force-7 gale. You couldn't look at this 'mo' and not feel a little bit less of a man than Kitchener himself. Kitchener's moustache is a classic example of the aloof, arrogant and patriarchal egotism required to goad young men to be machine-gunned to death in their tens of thousands. Imperial superiority and nutty Britishness oozes from the greased tip of every hair.

Ron Jeremy

He came from a good, middle-class Jewish family – his father was a physicist and his mother was a book editor – so few could have predicted that Ron Jeremy would end up being the most famous male porn star the world had ever seen (on video). Fat, hairy and with a moustache like a smear of dirt across his top lip, Jeremy was never going to cut it as a leading man in the traditional sense. While the young Ron Jeremy did graduate from college with a degree in theatre studies, it seems more likely that his ability to auto-fellate was more of a factor in his rise to pornographic infamy than his *Hamlet*. You don't need to have seen one of Ron's 2,000 hard-core films to know his tash. It's the moustache that every man fears will appear on his top lip when he grows one for the first time – a messy handful of hair that simply says 'porn star'.

GREAT BEARDED MEN THROUGH HISTORY

Chuck Norris

The official Chuck Norris facts website reports the following on the origins of the Norris beard: 'Wanna know how Chuck Norris grew his beard? He didn't, his beard grew him.' Carlos Ray 'Chuck' Norris is the star of *Walker, Texas Ranger*, the *Missing in Action* trilogy and countless other politically reactionary, explosively violent action movies that have made him a living legend. After serving in the United States Air Force, Norris began to climb the ladder of fame as a martial artist and even founded his own school, Chun Kuk Do, before moving to Hollywood – the rest is history. Whether it's fighting back to back with Bruce Lee, blasting rogue bikers at close range with a shotgun or twisting the head off an abusive Viet Cong prison guard, Chuck's closely trimmed beard has remained a constant. Norris' conservative, well-groomed face fuzz is the perfect complement to the compact power of his muscle-bound body and tough-guy attitude. Norris is a devout Christian and politically conservative in real life but his beard is bad to the bone.

Karl Marx

Despite the fact that he came up with his world-changing ideas in a small flat in north London, the writings of German philosopher and political theorist Karl Marx would form the basis of modern communism. Marx argued that the inequalities of capitalism would inevitably lead to its collapse. Just as capitalism had replaced feudalism, so he believed that socialism would eventually replace capitalism to create a classless society. It didn't turn out that way because socialism turned out to be rubbish unless you like horrible architecture and small, boxy cars, so they had to bring back capitalism again. Nonetheless, Marx's contribution to socio-economic theory remains immense. Also immense was the full beard he wore throughout his life, which contributed hugely to the room-filling gravitas of the man. Usually, theories involving the fall of society evolved in a public library in NW10 would be dismissed as the ravings of a mentalist, but when they came from a mind encased in 2lb of grey beard topped with a monstrous black storm cloud of a moustache, the world had to sit up and listen.

Jesus

Jesus of Nazareth, commonly known as Jesus H. Christ or simply Jesus, is the central figure of Christianity. Christians believe him to be the messiah that was foretold in the Old Testament and the Son of God who died and rose from the dead to provide salvation for all humankind. It would not be difficult to argue that – after Santa – he is probably the most famous beard man in the western world. But the iconic image of Jesus with his long hair and classic Ducktail is a relatively new one and it took several centuries for the image of the Son of Man to reach a standardised form in art. The image of a fully bearded 'hippie' Christ with long, straight hair and beard did not become the established norm until the sixth century in eastern Christianity, and much later in the west. Before that there were huge variations in the images of him, which tended to reflect the ethnic characteristics of the artist's local culture. Despite this, many Christians still believe that the commonly used image of Jesus – seen on the Shroud of Turin and in most Hollywood biopics – is historically accurate.

Abraham Lincoln

Abraham Lincoln served as the sixteenth – and some would say greatest – President of the United States. More importantly, he was the first president to wear a beard. If you doubt the esteem in which he is held, remember that his whiskered visage can still be found today on the five-dollar bill and carved into the stone of Mount Rushmore. The great liberator led the Union through the American Civil War and ended slavery, but he was born to a poor frontier family and was mostly self-educated. Despite his lack of formal schooling, he was an eloquent man and his Gettysburg Address is still the template for speeches about freedom to this day. Lincoln seems to have grown his iconic Chinstrap when he first achieved high office in his late forties. Despite some contemporary photographs being available, it is hard to define whether his face fluff was a Donegal or an Old Dutch – some pictures even show him with a Goatee. One thing is for certain, whatever Lincoln was rocking, it looked smokin' with a stove-pipe hat.

Che Guevara

The bearded image of a steely eyed Che Guevara looking heavenwards towards a new society is an immediately recognisable symbol of revolution. As such, its place on the walls of dingy, student bedrooms and market stall t-shirts has been assured forever. Ernesto Guevara, commonly known as

'Che', was an Argentine Marxist revolutionary and a major figure in the Cuban Revolution. As a medical student, Che had travelled by motorcycle throughout Latin America and was profoundly affected by the endemic poverty he witnessed there. He concluded that the region's economic inequalities were the result of capitalism and that the only remedy was world revolution. Having come to this earth-shattering conclusion, he grew a straggly Balbo, bought a beret and headed for Cuba. The success of the revolution in Cuba meant that in just a few short years, Che found global recognition in his struggle against 'the man' – which is just as well, because just eight years later 'the man' would execute him while trying to pull a similar stunt in Bolivia.

Santa Claus

Whether you believe in him or not, Santa Claus, also known as Saint Nicholas, Father Christmas, Kris Kringle or simply 'Santa', is *the* guy with a beard. Everyone's favourite toy philanthropist sports a full white, snowy chin rug worn long in all directions that covers most of his face and breaks only to reveal his red, rosy nose and cheeks, and the twinkling magic in his eyes. It's undeniable that this beard man has all the plays worked out. Let's add it up: a) everyone likes him; b) he's got a pimped-out, reindeer-powered ride that can fly; c) he works just one day a year (bringing gifts to the homes of the good children) for which he gets paid handsomely in sherry and mince pies. He doesn't even have to buy the toys he drops off as they've been made by elves in a secret non-union workshop. Basically, this bearded god spends 364 days of the year relaxing in his snowy hideaway in Lapland with Mrs Claus like some kind of rotund Bond villain. It's nice work if you can get it. No wonder he's always smiling.

Russell Brand

Russell Brand describes his flamboyant fashion sense as making him look like an 'S&M Willy Wonka'. A crucial part of this unique style is his wild bird's nest hairdo and pencil-thin beard. It's true that Brand is a multi-talented comedian, actor, columnist, author and presenter of radio and television who has appeared in several mainstream films, but there's no denying that each time he moves into a new field, the beard

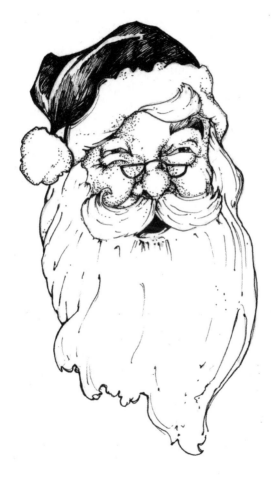

precedes him. Brand's clothes and hair are so intrinsic to his overall style that it's easy to forget that he's a dyed-in-the-wool beard man. Whether he's wearing it almost long enough to be a classic Boxed beard, or merely as a mischievous hint of carefully trimmed stubble, this unique facial statement is a very public symbol of his off-beat dandyism and on-going commitment to treading his own path.

Lord Alan Sugar

His beard may be greying, as he enters a dignified older age, but it still speaks volumes. Alan Michael Sugar, aka Lord Sugar, is a British entrepreneur and the short-tempered star of BBC TV's *The Apprentice*. Sugar started his business career boiling and selling beetroot on a council estate in the East End of London; now you can rent a corporate jet off him and he sits on a fortune estimated at £730 million. It's true there have been ups and downs in Sugar's phenomenal rise in business, notably his ill-fated chairmanship of Tottenham Hotspur football club, but throughout it all the wily cockney has kept his trademark face warmer with a smartly trimmed business beard. You could argue that the brevity of Sugar's face fuzz typifies his no-nonsense approach to business. However, the real reason for choosing this modest style may be that as a child Sugar had such profuse curly hair that he was nicknamed 'Mopsy' and, frankly, if he grew the beard any longer he'd look like a poodle.

John Lennon

Born to humble roots in Liverpool, John Lennon went on to conquer the world. As a member of the hugely popular band The Beatles, one half of the prodigious Lennon/McCartney song-writing partnership and as a solo artist, Lennon's creativity has been massively influential in popular music. Unlike his fellow mop-tops, Lennon's strong rebellious streak and art school roots could not be contained and they soon made themselves known through his extraordinary choices in facial hair. The Beatles may have risen to fame as clean-cut, suited and booted scousers, but all it took was a few million dollars and a couple of gallons of high-grade LSD for Lennon to freak out into the heavily bearded long hair of his later period. Lennon would go on to sport a heavy Walrus moustache, generous sideburns and even a Crew Cut and stubble combination, before finally returning to Earth some years later. Never has there been a more resonant example of the beard as a means of expressing individuality.

Charles Darwin

It is not often that you can say the work of one man has changed how we view the entire world, but the naturalist Charles Darwin did just that. In his seminal work *The Origin of the Species*, Darwin established the theory that all life on Earth had descended from a common ancestry and that the pattern of evolution was defined by a process he called natural selection, in which traits linked to survival were favoured. The book went a long way to explain the diversity of life on the planet but had the unfortunate side effect of undermining the role God might have played in creation. As a result, Darwin came in for a lot of flack in stridently Christian Victorian England, whose leading lights found it hard to accept that they had a common ancestor in the ape. A lifelong sideburn man, Darwin took the criticism badly and withdrew behind a full white beard

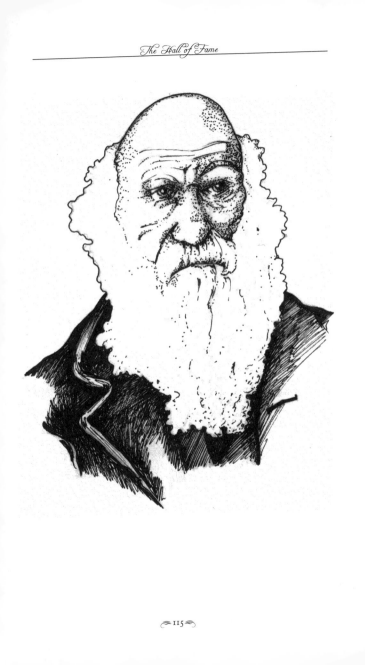

that can simply be described as epic. This practical example of follicular evolution turned a genius into a legend and added a terrifying air of gravitas to Darwin's look. It also made it a lot easier for nineteenth-century sketch writers to draw caricatures of him looking like a monkey – so everyone was a winner.

Grooming the Facial Fuzz

A WELL-GROOMED BEARD and moustache are like a lippy child – they will insist on growing and can become a terrible embarrassment unless they are cut down to size. How you choose to keep your beard or moustache in check is a matter of personal preference. Some people will only have this delicate work done professionally by a barber; others would rather die than let a stranger loose on their beloved facial fungus. Either way, a clean, well-groomed beard or moustache is the first step on the way to facial nirvana.

ESSENTIAL EQUIPMENT

Leonardo da Vinci didn't create the *Mona Lisa* with a tin of Dulux and a set of rollers from Homebase, so you shouldn't try to do the same with your beard. If you want to keep your beard or moustache looking great then you'll need the right kit. Every moustache aficionado and beard man will need the following in his bathroom:

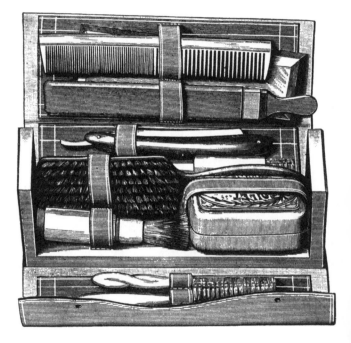

Scissors

If you decide to trim your beard or moustache primarily with scissors then it is worth investing in a decent pair of the kind used by professional barbers. They have longer, thinner blades which will afford you more flexibility when working with your whiskers and are sharp enough to cut the hair closely and cleanly without discomfort. If nothing else, investing in your own set of scissors will stop you getting it in the neck when your wife notices that her brand-new Kitchen Devils are blunt and covered in human topiary.

Comb

Just like the hair on your head, your beard and moustache will look less like birds have been nesting in it overnight if they are combed out in the morning. No matter what size your face is, you will need at least two combs in your armoury: a good wide-toothed comb for use on your beard, and a fine-toothed comb for the moustache – some speciality shops and barbers will sell small combs specifically designed for the purpose. A decent set of combs is essential not just for grooming but also trimming, should you choose to do it yourself.

Brush

While not an essential tool, a stiff bristle moustache brush can be a great way of sprucing up your hairy pal with minimum effort. Some moustache aficionados swear by their use when shaping and styling, particularly when they are working with stiff waxes.

Clippers or Trimmers

A good beard trimmer is an indispensable tool for the bearded man. These handy devices make it easy to keep beards well groomed and, as they almost always come with an adjustable trimming guide, you can set the height of the shears to handle any length of beard. Most trimmers will also allow you to remove this trimming guide for close work or to cut a border line. A set of trimmers is much more efficient and considerably easier to use than scissors. They will always give a consistent cut and do it in half the time – invaluable when you're half asleep and late for work.

Mirror

It might seem like a no-brainer, but a good-sized, well-lit wall mirror is indispensable for the grooming of beards and moustaches. Peering into a tiny vanity mirror that is no bigger than a porthole on a cross-Channel ferry will mean that you can't see what you're doing and your hard-grown glory will end up looking like a mess. Those who favour an ornate moustache design might also benefit from using a magnifying mirror for the close-up inspection of hard-to-see areas.

Styling Wax

Styling wax is a must if you have a moustache that requires some help to form its shape. It's generally sold in tubs, sticks or tubes and comes in a variety of weights which offer stronger or lighter holds. Some brands also offer coloured waxes to match your facial hair type. Most chemists carry a basic wax but you may need to visit a speciality shop or get on the internet to really shop around. It's probably best to try a

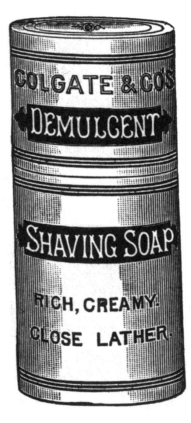

few different brands to see how they hold up with your particular style.

WASHING & TRIMMING BEARDS & MOUSTACHES

You may be sporting the world's greatest Imperial or a truly breathtaking Van Dyke, but if that morning's Rice Krispies are still lodged in it then you're going to spoil the effect. Keeping a well-groomed beard and moustache means that you must ensure they are clean. After all, you will literally be eating your dinner off it.

Washing your Beard or Moustache

Here is a ten-point guide to keeping your whiskers clean and kissable:

☞ Shampoo and condition your beard and moustache daily.
☞ Wet your face and rub in a good-quality shampoo.

☞ Make sure that you properly apply it to the hair follicles and massage gently down the face in a circular motion. This will help you clean your beard effectively and remove any dirt that might have collected in it.

☞ Rinse with clean water.

☞ Rub in a good-quality conditioner to soften the whiskers using the same method.

☞ Rinse again with clean water.

☞ Dry the beard with the help of a clean, dry towel.

☞ Don't press or rub your beard aggressively as this may cause irritation on your skin.

☞ Comb out your whiskers. Style as appropriate.

☞ Smile into the mirror. You look gorgeous, you handsome devil.

Trimming your Beard or Moustache

So you've put in all the hard work and have a sparkling clean face full of follicles. Now what? Your beard or moustache might look stylin' today, but if you don't put some effort into grooming, you will end up looking like a wino. Be warned

– there are only a couple of weeks of unchecked growth between looking like you should be piloting Concorde and looking like you should be selling *The Big Issue* outside Camden Town tube.

Here are a few easy steps to help you develop your trimming and styling skills:

Step 1: Get Tooled Up

Before you start you'll need the right gear. Decide whether to trim using scissors or a beard trimmer or both.

Step 2: Keep It Dry

Do not try to trim a wet beard or moustache. Wet hair is heavier and will hang longer. When it dries and retracts you may find you've trimmed too much.

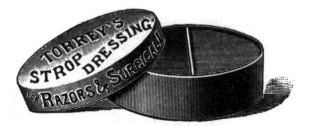

Step 3: Comb & Cut

To trim your moustache, first comb it straight down. Then use either the beard trimmer or scissors. Use the line of your lip as a template to cut along. Start in the middle and trim first towards one side of the mouth, then towards the other.

If you are using a comb and scissors, comb through the moustache and cut the hair on the outside of the comb. Perfecting this technique will take some practice but it is the only way to ensure you trim the hair evenly.

Depending on the style of your moustache, you may need to wet shave around the areas of growth.

If you have a beard, always start from the border of the beard and gradually trim into the internal areas. If you are adopting a particular style of beard then you can use the trimmer to help you craft a square or round border for the beard.

When working on the body of the beard, set your trimmer's adjustable trimming guide to a length you are comfortable with. When trimming, always move the beard trimmer vertically. You are looking for consistent length, so only trim off the longer and more unruly hairs.

Use the beard trimmer with the adjustable trimming guide removed to keep the neck line of your beard well defined and close crop the neck. Alternatively, you could carefully shave the lower portion of your neck.

Step 4: Easy Does It

When you are first starting out it is better to err on the side of caution. Cut a little rather than risk cutting too much.

Likewise with a beard trimmer, until you've mastered its use, it is best to keep the adjustable trimming guide set for a longer beard length at first.

Take your time. Rome wasn't built in a day and neither was a good-looking beard or moustache. Carelessness or lack of patience can ruin months of effort.

Step 5: Stay in Balance

To help maintain a balance between the two sides of your face, you may find it useful to start near the ear on one side and trim down to the chin. Then repeat on the other side.

Miscellaneous stray hairs can be removed using the beard trimmer with the adjustable trimming guide removed or with a wet razor.

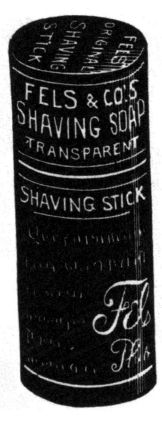

Step 6: Style & Preen

Gently stroke and smooth your whiskers into your desired style.

If you use styling wax, roll the wax across your fingers for a few seconds to allow it to soften before smoothing it on to your whiskers.

Manually create your style.

Take a step back and observe yourself in the mirror. Hark … is that the sound of ladies swooning?

Hints & Tips

- ☞ Keep a clean-shaved neck unless you want to look like a hamster.
- ☞ Facial hair is much coarser than the hair on your head. Soften it by using hair conditioner.
- ☞ Those with a full beard may find themselves getting dandruff. Regular use of decent conditioner should help with this.
- ☞ Massaging your beard and the area around it will keep the blood flowing and ensure healthy growth and soft, supple skin. Some eucalyptus or olive oil worked into the skin can help to strengthen the hair.

☞ When growing any facial hair, you will need to let your hair go unattended for about four weeks. Let a barber create an initial style for your beard the first time it is cut. You can follow his lines going forward.

☞ Your face is going to itch as you grow your beard out for the first time, so just keep washing and conditioning it to keep your whiskers soft and don't allow your skin to dry out underneath it.

☞ Don't pull out stray hairs, particularly on the neck. At best you'll end up looking like a plucked turkey, at worst they'll get infected.

☞ You can buy beard trimmers with and without cords and at a variety of different prices. In general, the cordless, rechargeable units from reputable brands are the most expensive but they're also the most reliable and the easiest to use.

☞ Don't believe the myths – shaving your beard will not make it grow back any faster or thicker than before.

WAXING & STYLING

The decision to use styling wax is a matter of personal choice between man and moustache. You may be one of those fortunate few who are blessed with hair that stays in shape on its own; however, most of us may need some waxy intervention. Be aware that there are also some practical considerations: assisted shaping may be the only way to achieve a particular style and it can help to keep hair out of the mouth with some longer styles. In general, you should use softer waxes for bushy moustaches, while thin, heavily styled creations will require a heavier wax to achieve and maintain definition.

Be Sparing

Less is always more when styling a moustache. Wax on the moustache will quickly become greasy and uncomfortable if you put too much on. Ideally you are looking to wax the ends of your soup-strainer to provide focus and shape, using the absolute minimum amount of product to keep the hairs in place.

Those with thicker growth may need some wax to train the hair in the centre of the lip to move out horizontally; however, try to use as little wax as possible here. There's a good chance it will get washed off when you drink anyway.

Applying Moustache Wax

Styling wax is usually supplied in a tub, stick or tube:

- For wax that comes in a tub, scoop some out and soften it by rolling it between your fingers for a few seconds before you work it into your moustache.
- When the wax is supplied in a tube it can be applied directly; however, it is usually better to squeeze some on to your fingers and work it into the whiskers manually.
- Wax that comes in the form of a stick can be applied directly to the hair.

In each case, work the wax into the whiskers from the centre outwards, then comb it through and shape the final style of the moustache with your fingers.

Removing Moustache Wax

All good waxes can be washed out easily with hot water and shampoo. You may find that some lighter waxes will simply be washed away or evaporate during the day due to humidity, perspiration or eating and drinking. If this is the case, they will need to be reapplied or you'll need to choose a heavier wax if you want to be in good shape come dinner time.

What to Look for in Moustache Wax

There is a surprising range of decisions to be made when looking for the wax to support your personal style. Mercifully, price is seldom a factor as the amount used day to day on a moustache is tiny, so whatever you buy should last a while.

You may like to consider the following:

Performance: Heavier waxes will be required for ornate and unusual styles, and especially when you're looking to keep the ends of your moustache in place. However, something big, beautiful and bushy needs little help.

Colour: Some waxes, like shoe polish, have an underlying colour in an attempt to blend seamlessly with the hair. Obviously you should not choose a colour that is very different from your natural hair colour. If you are unsure then choose neutral or uncoloured brands.

Perfume: The key factor in any styling wax that is overlooked at your peril is smell. This stuff is going to be sitting right under your hooter all day, so make sure you choose something that doesn't smell like a vet's waiting room.

Running Out of Wax

What do you do when you run out of wax? The short answer is go and buy some more. However, if you are really pushed there may be a solution. There have been many reports of wild and wonderful home-grown alternatives: Beeswax, Vaseline, gum-arabic, soap and even peanut butter, to name a few. There are also some enthusiasts who prefer to brew their own secret mixtures, with variable results.

A word of warning: don't think you can immediately raid your wife's dressing table if you come up short. In general, gels and hairsprays designed for the head can dry out the more sensitive hair and skin around the mouth and should be avoided.

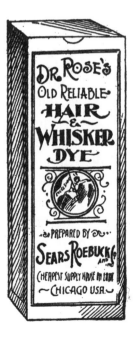

GET A GRIP: THREE LOST GROOMING TREASURES

A modern man might feel that it's one thing to take pride in his appearance and quite another to go over the top. However, our forefathers in the face fungus had no such qualms and chose to create several short-lived inventions to help with the styling and maintenance of their moustaches and beards.

Moustache Curlers

This is essentially a thin iron or steel bar similar to hair tongs which used heat to create a natural curl in the hair. Unfortunately, moustache curlers have not been manufactured for some years and so have not benefited from the technological advances enjoyed by their hair-styling cousins – automated temperature control, for example. If you find a moustache curler in an antique shop, you'll still need to heat it on the oven, which means every time you use it you'll run the risk of setting fire to your own tash.

Moustache Cup

The moustache cup was invented by British potter Harvey Adams in the 1860s. The cup has a semicircular ledge hidden inside with a small opening for liquids to pass through while guarding the moustache and keeping it dry. It is hard to see why this ingenious device is not still in production, but you may be able to pick one up online or in an antique shop.

Moustache Snood

The moustache snood or moustache band is a wide length of lightweight fabric cut to accommodate the nose. When worn around the head it covers the moustache at night to help keep its shape. A moustache snood is seen in dramatic action in Albert Finney's portrayal of Hercule Poirot in *Murder on the Orient Express*. You can pick one up on Amazon for twenty quid. Bear in mind that the modern lady may not share your dedication to good grooming so don't try it out on a first date.

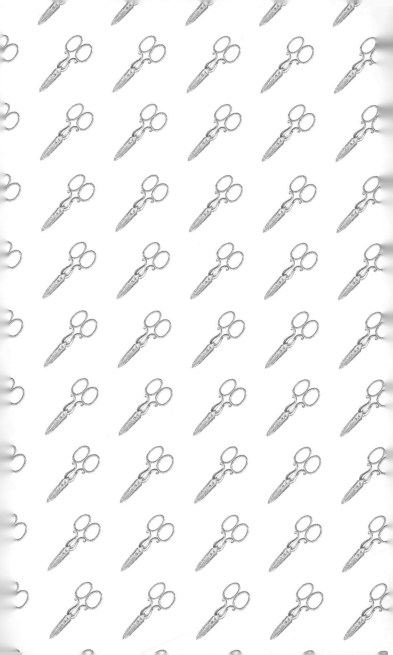

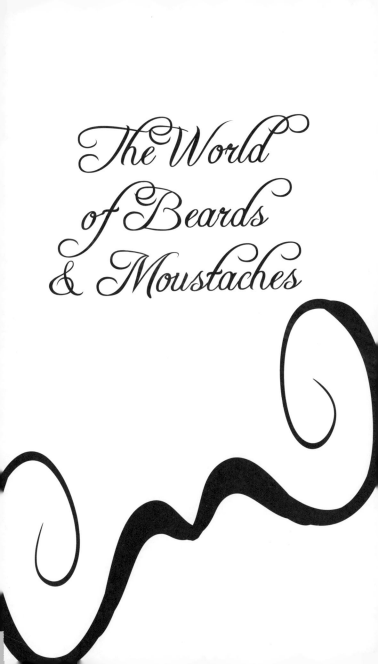

The World
of Beards
& Moustaches

QUOTES ABOUT BEARDS
& MOUSTACHES

OVE IT or hate it, facial hair can seldom be
ignored. As a result, lip muffs and nose
neighbours have often come under the scru-
tiny of history's greatest thinkers. Here's what the
great and the good have had to say about them:

There was an Old Man with a beard,
Who said, 'It is just as I feared! –
Two Owls and a Hen,
Four Larks and a Wren,
Have all built their nests in my beard!'
— Edward Lear, *Book of Nonsense*

Chins without beards deserve no honour.
— Proverb

Being kissed by a man who didn't wax his
moustache was like eating an egg without salt.
— Rudyard Kipling

There is always a period when a man with a beard shaves it off. This period does not last. He returns headlong to his beard.

> – Jean Cocteau

He that hath a beard is more than a youth, and he that hath no beard is less than a man.

> – William Shakespeare

I've grown this moustache which saves me from having to glue on one every day in the heat.

> – Keith Carradine

In England and America, a beard usually means that its owner would rather be considered venerable than virile; on the continent of Europe, it often means that its owner makes a special claim to virility.

> – Rebecca West, *The Thinking Reed*

Since I have dealt in suds, I could never discover more than two reasons for shaving; the one is to get a beard, the other is to get rid of one.

> – Henry Fielding

Don't point that beard at me, it might go off.
— Groucho Marx

All the power is with the sex that wears the beard.
— Molière

Upon shaving off one's beard: 'The scissors cut the long-grown hair; the razor scrapes the remnant fuzz. Small-jawed, weak-chinned, bug-eyed, I stare at the forgotten boy I was.'
— John Updike

Why is the King of Hearts the only one that hasn't a moustache?
— James Branch Cabell

A man without a moustache is like a cup of tea without sugar.
— English Proverb

There are two kinds of people in this world that go around beardless — boys and women — and I am neither one.
— Greek Saying

There are three kinds of man you must never trust: a man who hunts south of the Thames, a man who has soup for lunch; and a man who waxes his moustache.

> – Sir James Richards

When I went to the Olympics, I had every intention of shaving the moustache off, but I realized I was getting so many comments about it – and everybody was talking about it – that I decided to keep it.

> – Mark Spitz

A woman with a beard looks like a man. A man without a beard looks like a woman.

> – Afghan Saying

BEARD & MOUSTACHE RECORDS

Did you know that there are between 10,000 and 20,000 hairs on a man's face? While this is a pretty impressive fact, if you really want to get into the record books then it's not the number but what you do with them that counts. Below are some examples of people who have gone the extra mile with their facial hair.

Longest Moustache

The world's longest moustache belongs to India's Ram Singh Chauhan. The 54-year-old tour guide from Rajasthan became a tourist attraction himself when his immense Chin Fork was measured at a very respectable 4.29m (14ft).

Largest Group of People with Moustaches in One Place

The largest gathering of people with moustaches is 1,131. The record was set when fans of the Minnesota Wild hockey team and the Tom Selleck fan club came together at the Wild stadium to set the new world record for Movember – a global movement where men grow moustaches to raise money for testicular cancer. The previous world record was just 151, established by the fans of the Partick Thistle football club in Glasgow.

Longest Beard

Currently, the world's longest beard measures 2.37m (7ft 9in) and belongs to Sarwan Singh of

Canada. This would be a truly impressive growth were it not for the fact that the longest beard ever measured belonged to Hans Langseth of Norway. At the time of his death in 1927, it hung proud at an incredible 5.65m (18ft 6in).

Greatest Weight Lifted by a Beard

The greatest weight lifted with a human beard is 63.2kg (139.33lb). Lithuanian nutcase Antanas Kontrimas achieved the incredible feat on 16 September 2007 when he lifted a girl 10cm (3.93in) off the ground on the set of a *Guinness World Records* special in Beijing. Nevertheless, his impressive feat may be topped by the pure insanity of Ismael Rivas Falcon of Spain, who pulled a train weighing 2,753.1kg (6,069lb) over a distance of 10m (32.8ft) with his beard in Madrid on 15 November 2001.

Longest Beard Chain

What is a beard chain? It's simply a lovely chain of men linked together by their beards. The world's longest consisted of twenty participants and measured 19.05m (62ft 6in). This heart-warming event was achieved by the members of

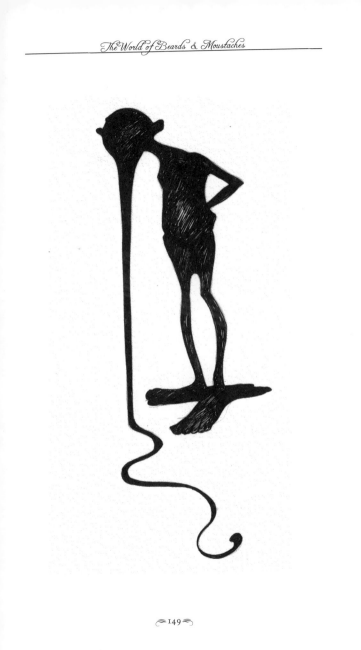

the *Verband Deutscher Bartclubs e. V* in Amberg, Germany, on 2 December 2007.

Best Moustache Stroker

Every man that wears a tash! The average man with a moustache will touch his lady tickler an amazing 760 times in any twenty-four-hour period.

BEARDS & MOUSTACHES IN NATURE

Facial hair may be found on some of the most handsome alive today, but this kind of commitment to style is not exclusive to the human race – it is also a feature of the world of beasts. Whether they're swinging from a tree in a rainforest or hiding beneath a rock in a fast-moving stream, our zoological friends still want to look their best and some facial hair can make all the difference. Mother Nature has always been ahead of the game on this one and we were forced to assess goats, collies and even the bearded tit in our quest to identify the best beards in the wild. We can all grab a little inspiration from our countdown of the top five face-dos from the animal kingdom.

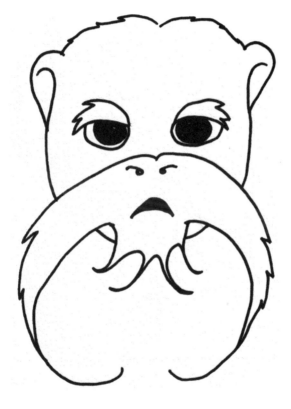

5. Moustached Tamarin

The tamarin is a squirrel-sized monkey from the family Callitrichidae in the genus *Saguinus*. Different tamarin species vary considerably in appearance, ranging from nearly all black to mixtures of black, brown and white, but all have a marvellous bushy moustache that is common to the variants of this species and Mexican bandits. You can find them right across southern Central America, where they reside in the tropical rainforests of the Amazon basin. Tamarins are omnivores. This means that they eat fruit as well as spiders, insects and eggs – so let's hope they also have tiny monkey combs to keep their cookie dusters clear of unsightly debris.

4. The Schnauzer

Schnauzers are friendly and fun-loving dogs that originated in Germany in the fifteenth and sixteenth centuries. They may be small in stature, but when it comes to showing off with the facials, the Schnauzer goes big. Even its name is derived from *Schnauze*, the German word for 'snout', because of the dog's distinctive grey face fuzz. The word 'Schnauzer' can also mean 'moustache'

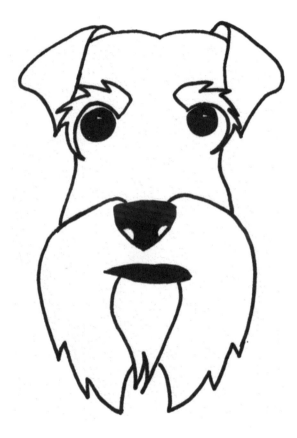

in German. Without splitting hairs, it might be more accurate to define the word as 'circle beard', as the Teutonic terriers tend to sport an impressively groomed beard and moustache combination.

3. The Catfish

Catfish are a remarkable diverse group of ray-finned fish which range in size and behaviour. The heaviest and longest reside in the Mekong delta in South East Asia, while the smallest, known as Candiru, are little more than tiny parasites. What they all have in common, however, is a stonker of a tash. These prominent barbels are thought to resemble a cat's whiskers – hence the name; in fact, they look more like magnificently styled waxed English moustaches. The larger breeds of catfish are commonly farmed or fished in open waters for food – although it's very possible they might be better deployed as models in the barber's shop.

2. Bearded Dragon

More commonly known as bearded dragons to reflect their proud dangling Goatees, *Pogona* are actually a genus of lizards that contain seven different species. These scaly creatures live in the semi-desert regions and dry open woodlands of Australia and are enthusiastic climbers, spending time on branches and in bushes, and are even found squatting on fence posts. Like their human Goatee-wearing counterparts, bearded dragons are pretty bohemian creatures. They are primarily active only in the evening and choose to spend their mornings and afternoons basking on rocks doing nothing – one assumes nursing one hell of a hangover from the night before.

1. The Lion

He's the daddy of all meat-eaters with a roar that could loosen your bowels from a hundred paces, so it's no surprise that the lion's bearded face can be found in cave paintings from as early as the Upper Palaeolithic period. Typically an inhabitant of the grassy savannah of sub-Saharan Africa, the lion (aka the king of the beasts) is one of the four big cats in the genus *Panthera* and the number one beard-wearer in nature. While most female lions live for around fourteen years in the wild, the male lion is so hard

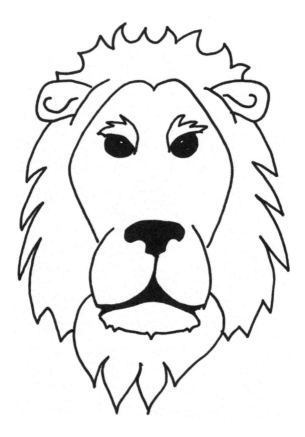

that he seldom lives longer than ten as a result of the injuries he sustains from continual aggro. When he's not fighting, he's chilling or eating meat – no bap, no lecture, no fries, just meat. It's perfectly understandable that such a hard nut would go for something special, and the lion's highly distinctive mane hinges around nature's most epic chin curtain. We salute you, sir!

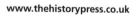 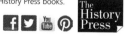